Marwa Gargouri
Héla Gargouri

Assessment of nursing knowledge about hepatitis C

Marwa Gargouri
Héla Gargouri

Assessment of nursing knowledge about hepatitis C

Nursing knowledge of chronic hepatitis C: epidemiology, modes of transmission, treatment and prevention

ScienciaScripts

Imprint

Any brand names and product names mentioned in this book are subject to trademark, brand or patent protection and are trademarks or registered trademarks of their respective holders. The use of brand names, product names, common names, trade names, product descriptions etc. even without a particular marking in this work is in no way to be construed to mean that such names may be regarded as unrestricted in respect of trademark and brand protection legislation and could thus be used by anyone.

Cover image: www.ingimage.com

This book is a translation from the original published under ISBN 978-620-6-71525-2.

Publisher:
Sciencia Scripts
is a trademark of
Dodo Books Indian Ocean Ltd. and OmniScriptum S.R.L publishing group

120 High Road, East Finchley, London, N2 9ED, United Kingdom
Str. Armeneasca 28/1, office 1, Chisinau MD-2012, Republic of Moldova, Europe
Printed at: see last page
ISBN: 978-620-7-77351-0

CONTENTS

INTRODUCTION 2

MATERIALS AND METHODS 3

ANALYSIS AND RESULTS 6

DISCUSSION 28

CONCLUSION 52

BIBLIOGRAPHY 53

APPENDIX 56

INTRODUCTION

Hepatitis C is a chronic infection of the liver caused by a virus that is transmitted mainly by blood. While 20% of those infected recover spontaneously, hepatitis C becomes a chronic disease in 80% of those infected.of cases. If the disease is not diagnosed and treated in time, it can lead to cirrhosis and even liver cancer. There is as yet no vaccine to protect against it [1].

Hepatitis C virus (HCV) infection affects 3% of the world's population. In Tunisia, according to recent statistics, its prevalence is 1.6% in the general population, with a South-North gradient. Prevalence is 0.26% in the south and 2.9% in the north-west (level B) [2].

Nowadays, with the number of cases of chronic hepatitis C on the rise, these infections have become a cause for concern. In addition, healthcare professionals have experienced a higher risk of HCV infection than the general population. For this reason, we focused on these workers to assess their knowledge of chronic hepatitis C, its various modes of transmission, available treatments and preventive measures.

MATERIALS AND METHODS

1. Search quote :

This is a descriptive cross-sectional study conducted among nurses at the University Hospital of Gabès, with the aim of assessing nurses' knowledge of hepatitis C: its epidemiology, modes of transmission, treatments and preventive measures.In the course of this study, the members questioned responded in the following ways to our questionnaire.

2. Environment and period of study

This study was carried out at the University Hospital of Gabès from the month of February until March 2023.

The services included in my study were the following:

- ► Men's surgery
- ► Women's surgery
- ► Cardiology
- ► Dialysis
- ► Gynaecology
- ► Maternity ward
- ► Emergencies
- ► General medicine
- ► Infectious Diseases
- ► Pneumology
- ► Paediatrics
- ► Resuscitation

3. Study population :

In terms of this study, we have chosen to study a population of 80 health workers practising their profession at the University Hospital of Gabes between the departments most exposed to being in contact with HCV-infected patients confirmed or suspected of being infected with HCV with this distribution:

▶ Men's surgery: 10

▶ Paediatrics: 10

▶ Gynaecology: 8

▶ Emergencies: 7

▶ Maternity: 7

▶ Infectious diseases: 7

▶ Dialysis: 6

▶ Cardiology: 6

▶ Resuscitation: 6

▶ Pneumology: 5

▶ Women's surgery: 4

▶ General medicine: 4

4. Inclusion and exclusion criteria :

a. Inclusion criteria

√ Nurses working in Male and Female Surgery, Cardiology, Dialysis, Gynaecology and Maternity, Emergency, General Medicine, Infectious Diseases, Pneumology, Paediatrics and Intensive Care.

√ There are two types of nurse.

√ Nurses who work mornings, afternoons and nights.

√ Nurses of different ages.

b. Exclusion criteria :

✓ The refusal declared by certain healthcare staff.

✓ Staff working in other departments.

✓ Absence of certain staff during our study period.

5. Measuring instrument :

The data were collected using an anonymous questionnaire consisting of 29 questions targeted at 80 nurses working at the University Hospital of Gabès.

6. Data collection process :

I went to the 12 departments to inform potential staff about the study (context and objectives) and then distributed the questionnaire to those who agreed to take part.Each employee spent an average of 15 minutes answering the various parts of the questionnaire.

7. Data capture and analysis :

The data is collected manually. The data were entered and analysed using computer equipment (PC), typed in Microsoft Office Word 2010 and processed using Microsoft Excel 2010.The results were presented in graphical form.

8. Difficulties encountered :

Some nurses refused to answer the questionnaire, while others replied. carelessly.

ANALYSIS AND RESULTS

I. Characteristics of the participating nurse :

1. Breakdown of nurses by department :

Table 1: Breakdown of nurses by department

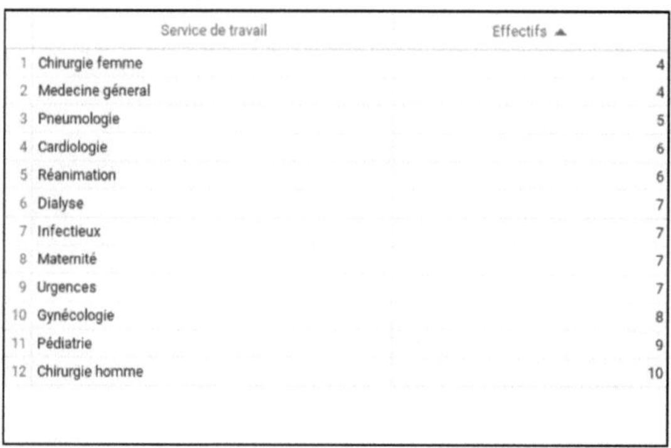

	Service de travail	Effectifs ▲
1	Chirurgie femme	4
2	Medecine géneral	4
3	Pneumologie	5
4	Cardiologie	6
5	Réanimation	6
6	Dialyse	7
7	Infectieux	7
8	Maternité	7
9	Urgences	7
10	Gynécologie	8
11	Pédiatrie	9
12	Chirurgie homme	10

The staff interviewed in our population were spread across 12 departments. The majority of participants worked in paediatrics and male surgery (12.5% each).

2. Breakdown of nurses by age :

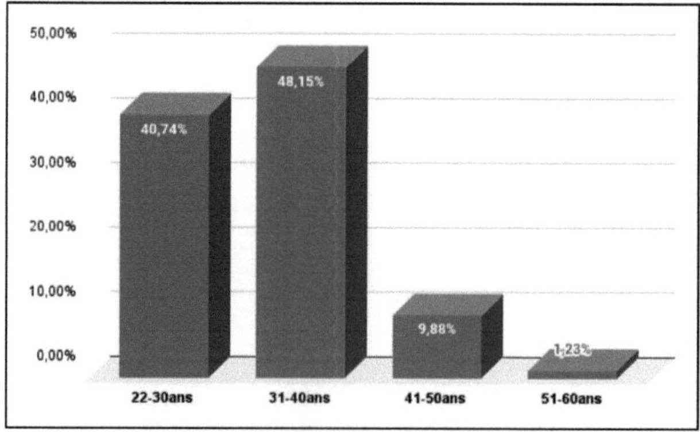

Figure 1: Breakdown of nurses by age

The results of this graph show that almost half of our population is in the 31-40 age group (48.15%).

3. Breakdown of nurses by gender :

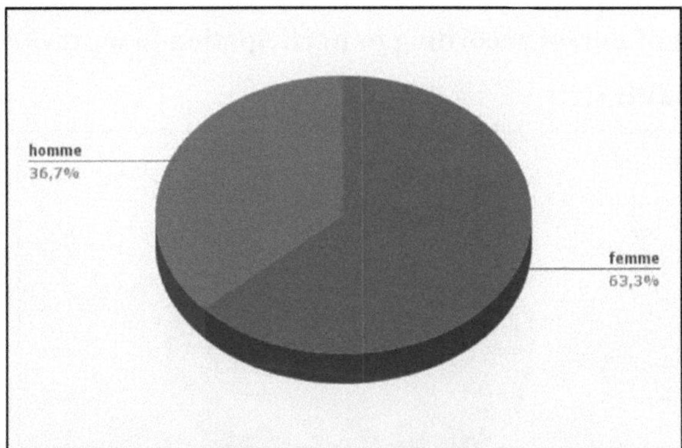

Figure 2: Breakdown of nurses by gender

These results show that the majority of the population studied is women (63%).

4. Breakdown of nurses by length of service :

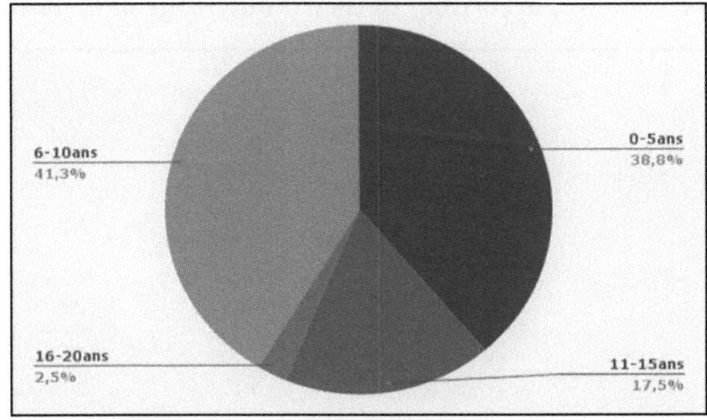

Figure 3: Breakdown of nurses by length of service

Of the subjects interviewed, the majority (42%) had been with the company for between 6 and 10 years.

II. **General knowledge about hepatitis** C :

1. Distribution of nurses according to participation in a previous training course on hepatitis C:

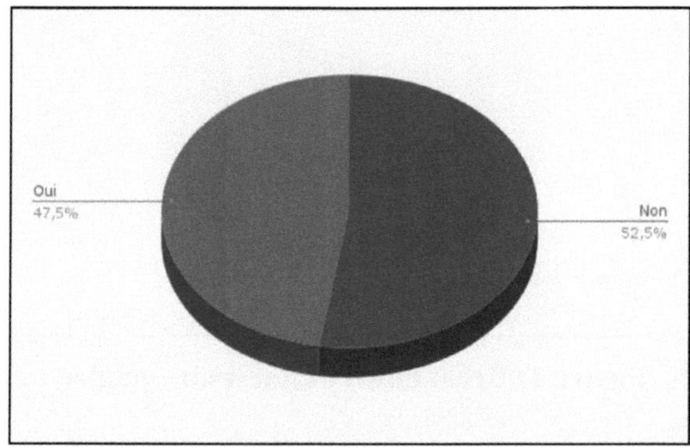

Figure 4: Distribution of nurses according to previous training on hepatitis C

More than half of the nurses questioned (52%) had not participated in a previous training in hepatitis C.

2. Distribution of nurses according to their knowledge of hepatitis C :

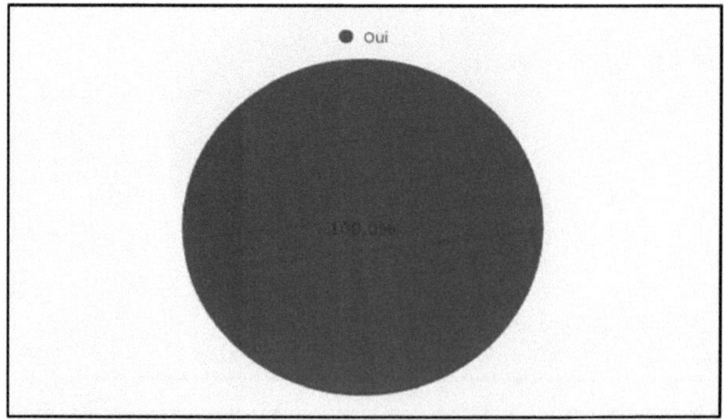

Figure 5: Distribution of nurses according to knowledge of hepatitis C

All the nurses interviewed knew the definition of hepatitis C.

3. Distribution of nurses according to knowledge of the agent responsible for hepatitis C:

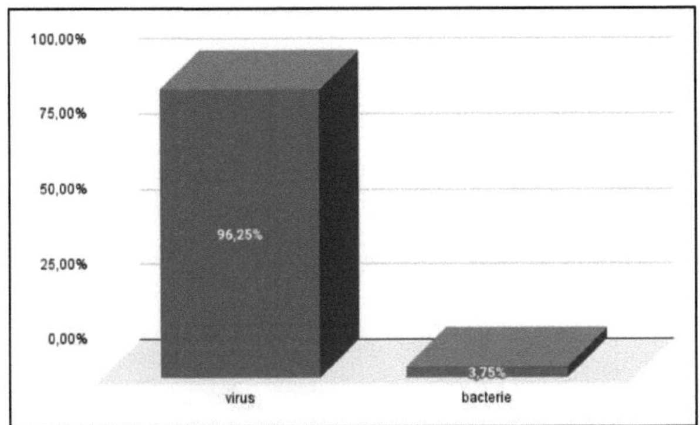

Figure 6: Distribution of nurses according to knowledge of the Agent responsible for hepatitis C

The majority of the population (96%)knew thatthe agent responsible for hepatitis C is a virus.

4. Distribution of nurses according to knowledge of methods of transmission of hepatitis C :

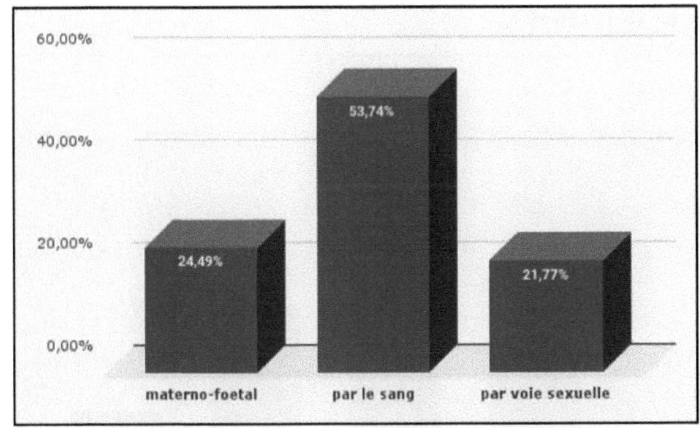

Figure 7: Distribution of nurses according to knowledge of modes of transmission of hepatitis C

According to the responses collected, the most frequent mode of HCV transmission was blood contamination (53.74%).

5. Distribution of nurses according to knowledge of resources transmission of hepatitis in healthcare settings :

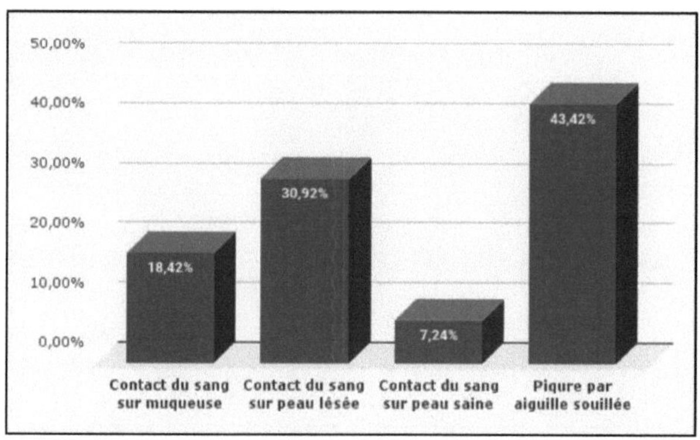

Figure 8: Distribution of nurses according to their knowledge of how hepatitis is transmitted in the healthcare setting

According to the majority of nurses questioned, the main means of transmission of hepatitis C in the healthcare environment were needlesticks (43.4%) and contact of blood with injured skin (30.9%).

6. Distribution of nurses according to their knowledge of the possible complications of hepatitis C :

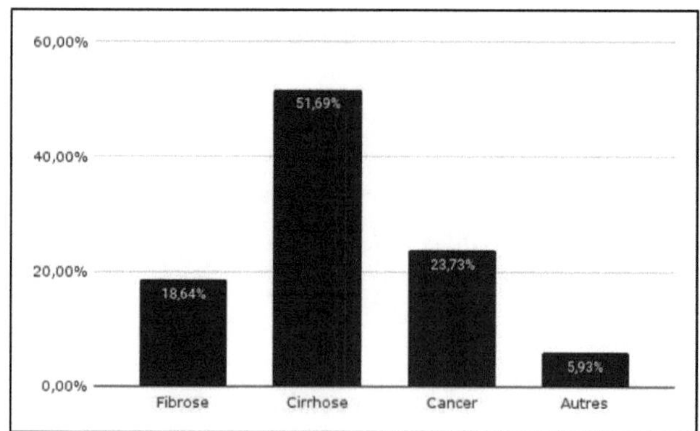

Figure 9: Distribution of nurses according to their knowledge of the possible complications of hepatitis C

More than half the population studied (51.7%) responded that cirrhosis is the major complication of hepatitis C, followed by liver cancer (23.73%).

7. Distribution of nurses according to knowledge of resources to prevent hepatitis C :

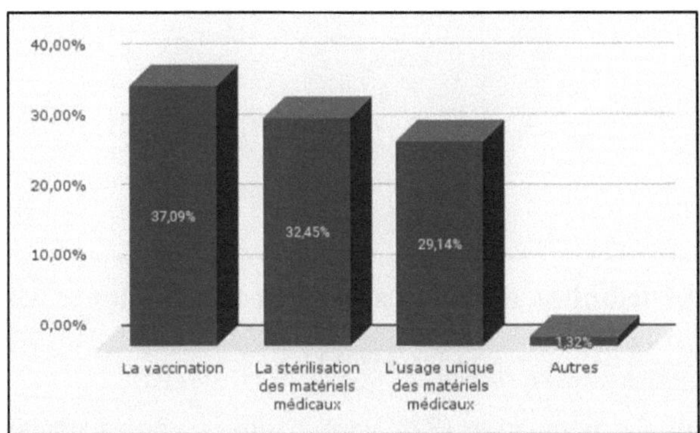

Figure 10: Distribution of nurses according to knowledge of hepatitis C prevention methods

The majority of staff questioned (37%) responded that vaccination is a means of preventing hepatitis C, while 32.4% chose sterilisation of medical equipment.

8. Distribution of nurses according to compliance with practices preventive measures against hepatitis C :

1.1.Distribution of nurses according to compliance with washing hands :

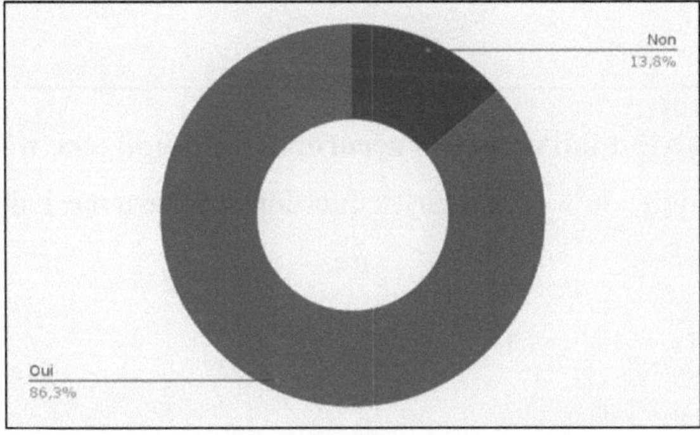

Figure 11: Distribution of nurses according to compliance with hand washing In our study, most nurses(86%) complied with hand washing.

1.2. Distribution of nurses according to compliance with wearing gloves :

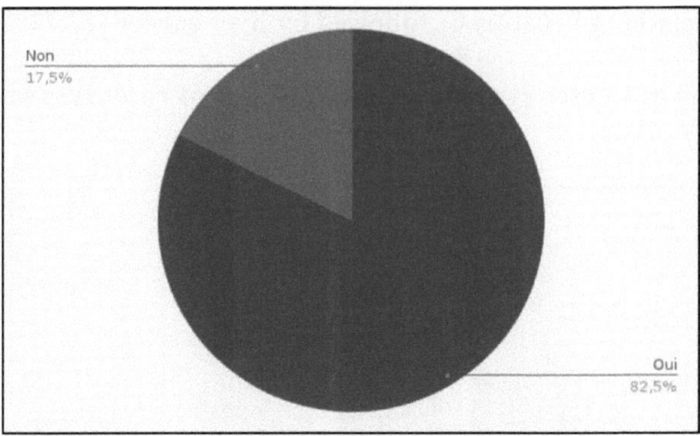

Figure 12: Distribution of nurses according to compliance with wearing gloves

The majority of the population (82%) wore gloves when carrying out nursing care.

1.3.Distribution of nurses according to compliance with mask wear :

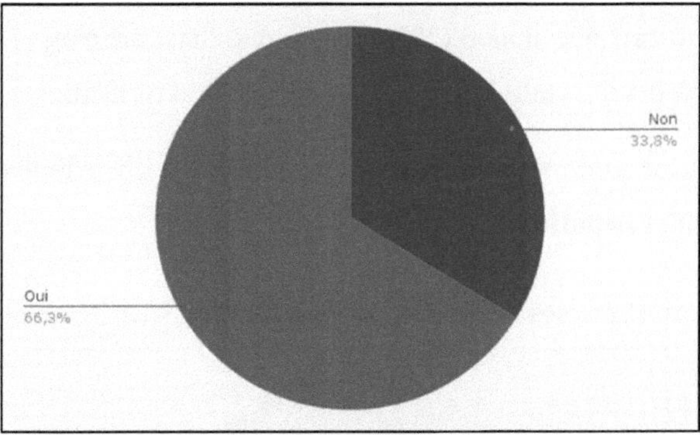

Figure 13: Distribution of nurses according to compliance with wearing a mask In our study, 66% of the nurses questioned wore a mask during nursing care.

1.4. Distribution of nurses according to compliance with wearing a smock :

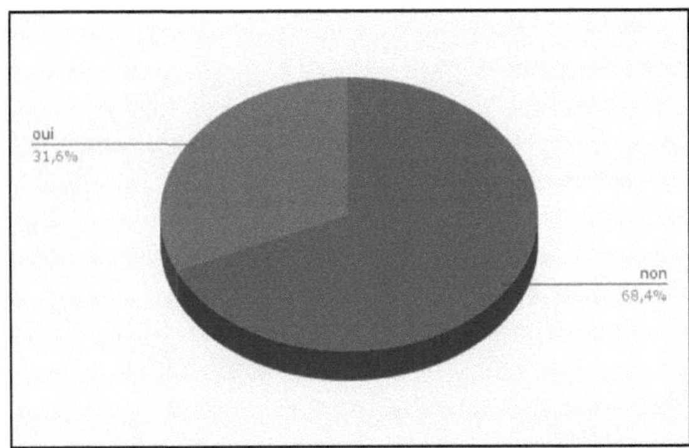

Figure 14: Distribution of nurses according to compliance with the wearing of smocks Most staff (68%) reported that they do not comply with the wearing of smocks in the care environment.

1.5. Breakdown of nurses by the compliance of not recapping needles after use:

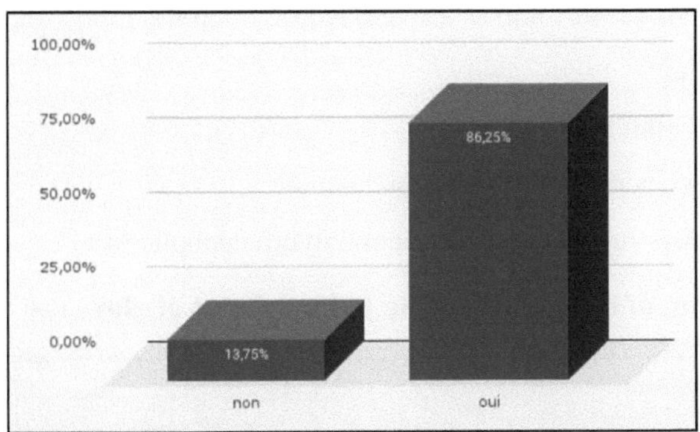

Figure 15: Distribution of nurses by compliance with not recapping needles after use

The majority of the population (86.25%) statedthat they respectnot recapping needles after use.

9. Distribution of nurses according to knowledge of hand cleaning :

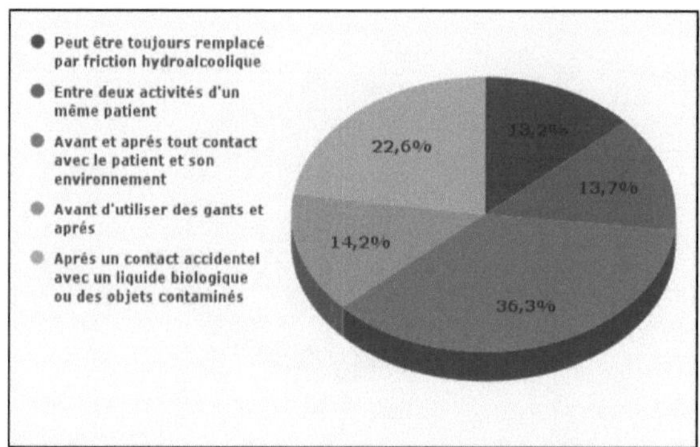

Figure 16: Distribution of nurses according to hand-cleaning knowledge

■According to 36.3% of staff, hands should be cleaned before and after any contact with the patient and their environment.

■22.6% of nurses felt that hands should be cleaned after each accidental contact with biological fluids or objects contaminants.

■A percentage of 41% of nurses are divided between the following indications for hand washing:

► Before and after using gloves

► Between two activities for the same patient

► Can be always replaced with a friction hydroalcoholic rub

10. Distribution of nurses according to knowledge of glove use :

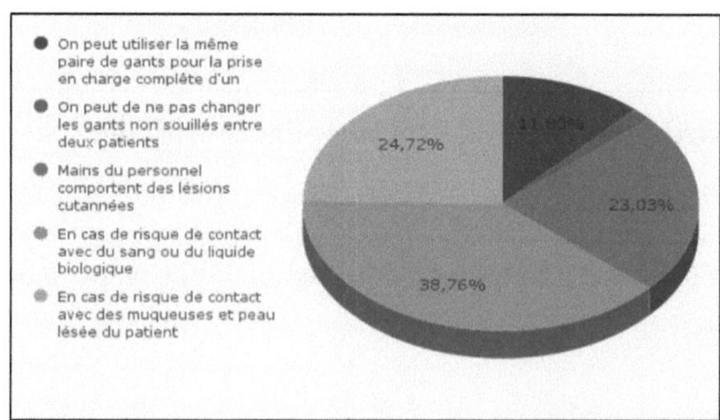

Figure 17: Distribution of nurses by knowledge of glove use

According to most of the population surveyed (38.76%), gloves should be worn when there is a risk of contact with mucous membranes or injured skin, while 6% felt that unsoiled gloves should not be changed between patients.

11. Distribution of nurses according to knowledge of overblouse use :

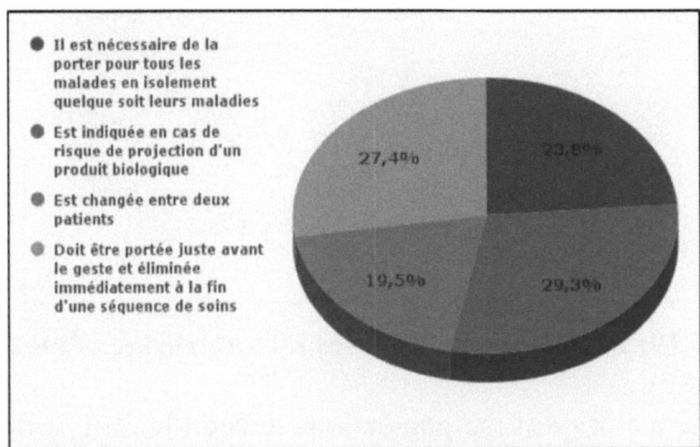

Figure 18: Distribution of nurses according to knowledge of overblouse use

• According to 29.3% of the population surveyed, overblanketing is indicated in cases of risk of splashing a biological liquid.

• According to 27.4% of nurses questioned, the overblouse should be worn just before the nursing procedure and removed immediately afterwards.

• For 23.8% of nurses, it is necessary to wear an overblouse for all patients in isolation, whatever their illness.

• According to 19.5% of staff, the gown must be changed between patients.

12. Distribution of nurses according to knowledge of mask use :

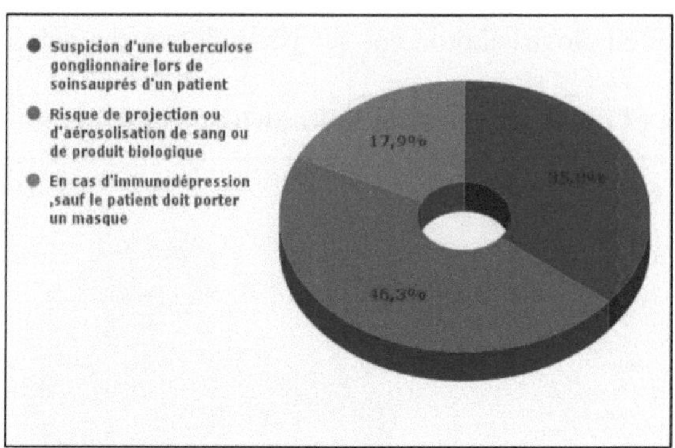

Figure 19: Distribution of nurses by knowledge of mask use

According to the majority of the population studied (46.3%), wearing a mask is recommended when there is a risk of spraying or aerosolisation of blood or biological products.

III. Evaluation of attitudes and practices towards risk of hepatitis c :

1. Distribution of nurses according to knowledge of contaminants handled by nurses :

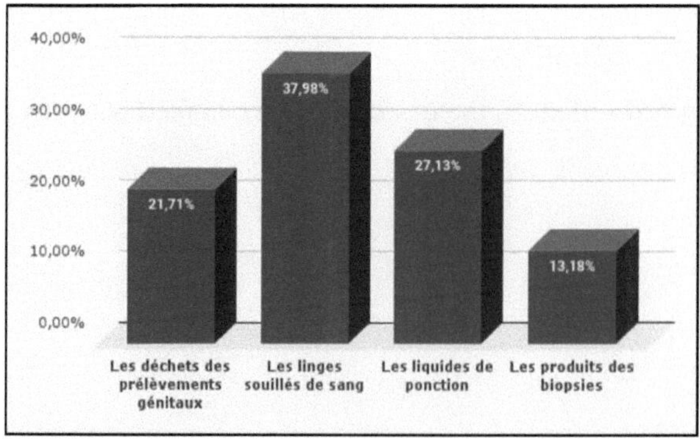

Figure 20: Distribution of nurses by knowledge of contaminants

According to most of the nurses questioned (38%), the contaminating products they handled were blood-stained cloths, followed by puncture fluids (27%).

2. Distribution of nurses according to their knowledge of contaminated medical devices handled by nurses :

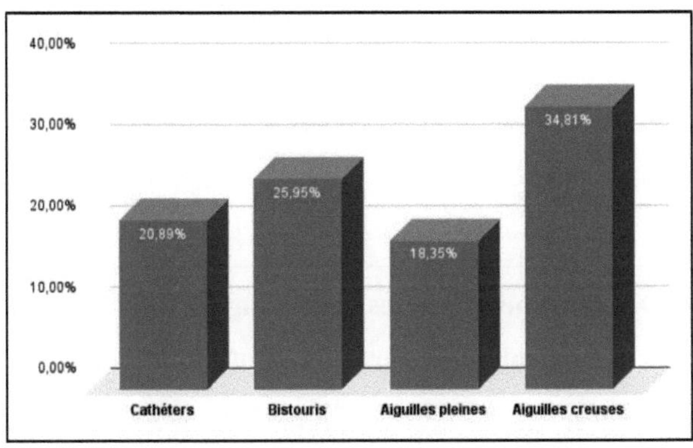

Figure 21: Distribution of nurses by knowledge of contaminated medical devices

According to 34.8% of nurses, the contaminating medical equipment was hollow needles.

■ 26% of respondents felt that the contaminating materials handled were scalpels.

■ 21% handled catheters, which may be contaminated

■ According to 18.3% of staff, the contaminating materials were solid needles.

3. Breakdown of nurses by knowledge of possible medical procedures for contamination:

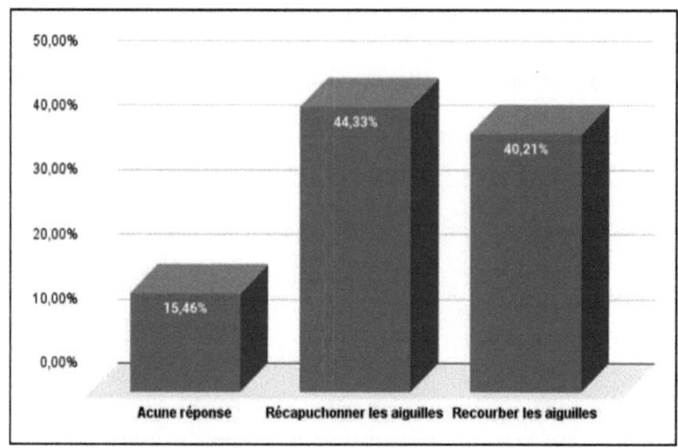

Figure 22: Distribution of nurses according to knowledge of possible medical procedures for contamination

According to 44% of people questioned, recapping needles is the most contaminating action.

4. Distribution of nurses according to compliance with protective and preventive measures :

1.1. Distribution of nurses according to compliance with personal protective equipment :

A.Distribution of nurses according to compliance with wearing of gowns :

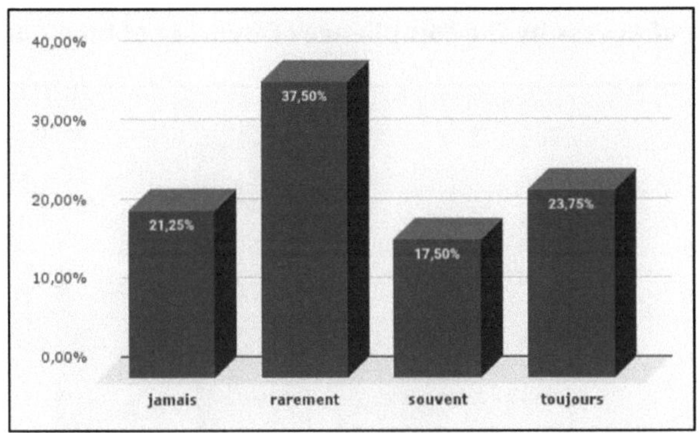

Figure 23: Distribution of nurses by compliance with the wearing of gowns

The majority of the population rarely wears a smock w h i l e carrying out their work. work (37.5%).

B. Breakdown of nurses by the compliance of wearing helmets during work:

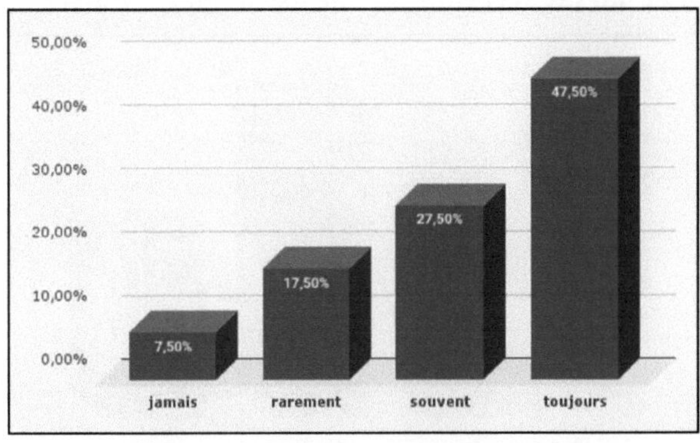

Figure 24: Distribution of nurses according to compliance with wearing helmets during work

Mostrespondents (47.5%) always wearhelmets at work.

C.Breakdown of nurses by the compliance of wearing of bibs during work:

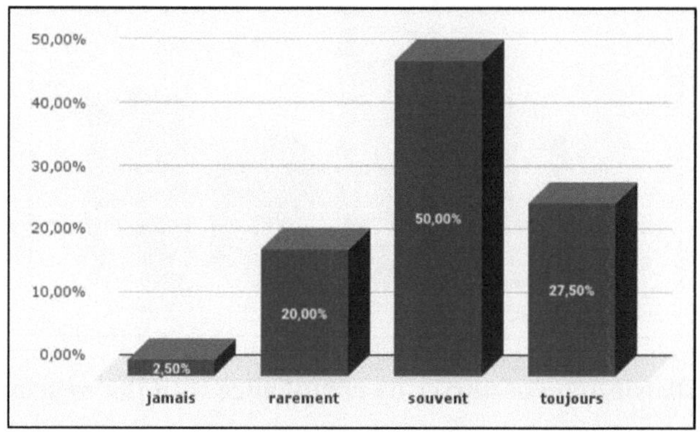

Figure 25: Distribution of nurses according to compliance with wearing bibs during labour

Half the population wears bibs at work.

D.Distribution of nurses according to the use of gloves during work :

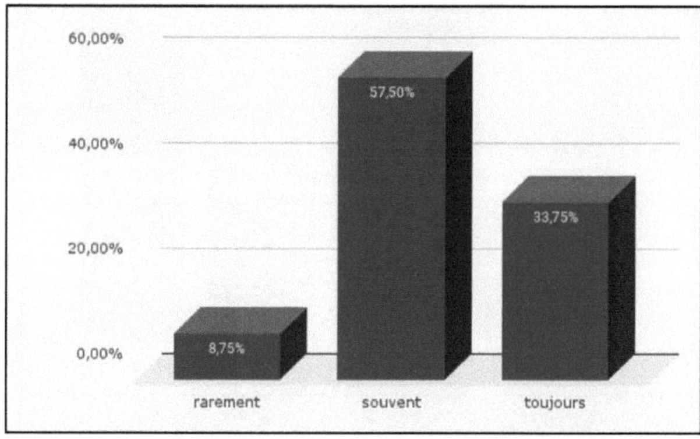

Figure 26: Distribution of nurses by wearing gloves at work

The majority of the population (57.5%) often wear gloves at work.

1.2. Distribution of nurses according to hand disinfection

A. Distribution of nurses according to hand disinfection with soap or 12° bleach diluted 1:10:

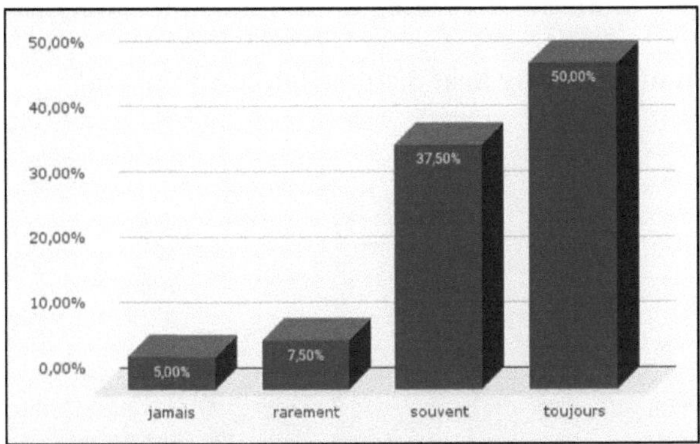

Figure 27: Distribution of nurses according to hand disinfection with soap or bleach at 12° diluted 1:10

Half of the population studied disinfect their hands with soap or 12° bleach diluted 1:10.

B. Distribution of nurses according to hand disinfection with alcohol 70° or other antiseptic:

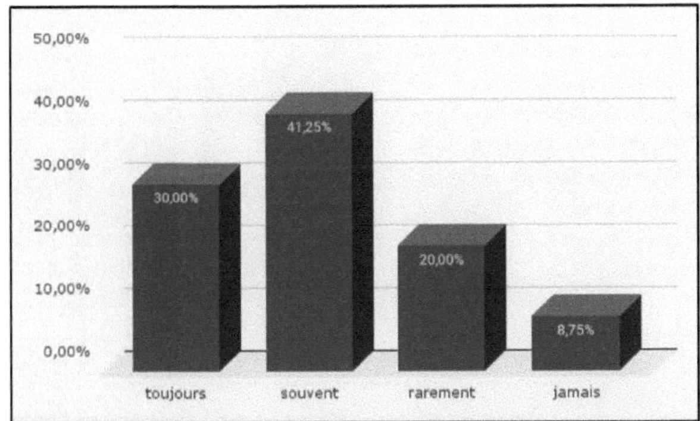

Figure 28: Distribution of nurses according to hand disinfection with 70° alcohol or other antiseptic

Most respondents (41.25%) often disinfect their hands with alcohol at 70° or another antiseptic such as dakin.

1.3. Distribution of nurses according to equipment disinfection :

A. Distribution of nurses by heat disinfection of equipment :

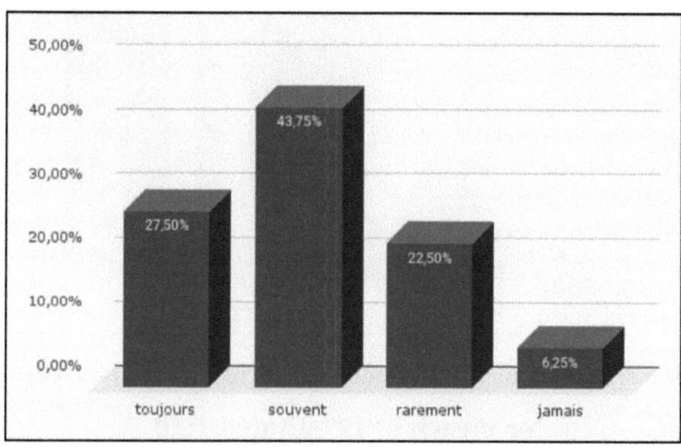

Figure 29: Distribution of nurses by heat disinfection of equipment

- Most of the population studied (43.7%) often disinfects equipment using heat

B. Distribution of nurses according to disinfection of equipment with soap :

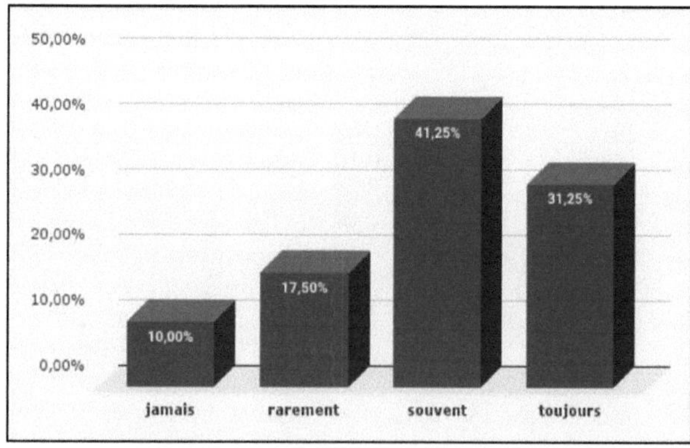

Figure 30: Distribution of nurses according to disinfection of equipment with soap

According to our survey, 41.25% of respondents indicated that they often disinfect equipment with soap.

C.Distribution of nurses according to disinfection of equipment with bleach:

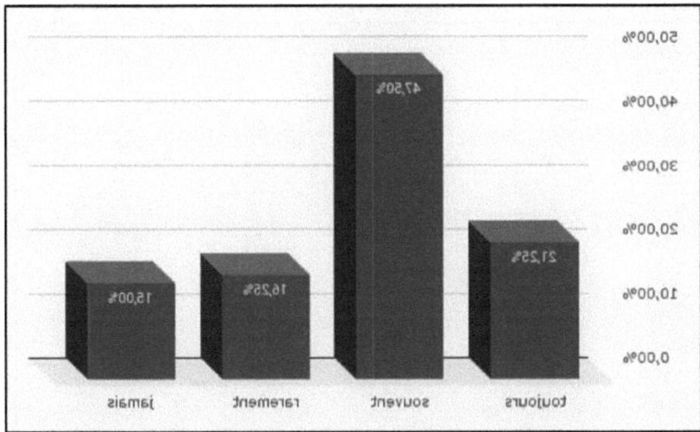

Figure 31: Distribution of nurses according to disinfection of equipment with bleach

The majority of nurses (47.5%) questioned often disinfect equipment with bleach.

1.4. Distribution of nurses according to workplace disinfection :

A. Distribution of nurses by product used to disinfect workplaces :

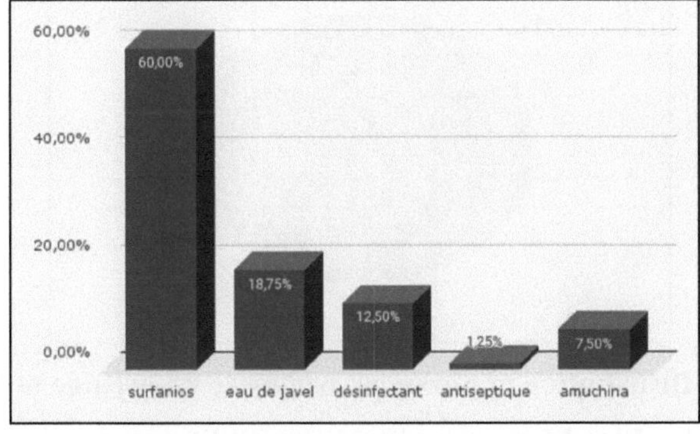

Figure 32: Distribution of nurses by product used to disinfect workplaces

According to the majority of the population (60%), surfanios was the main product used for disinfecting workplaces, while only 1% disinfected their workplaces with an antiseptic.

D. Distribution of nurses according to frequency of disinfection of workplaces :

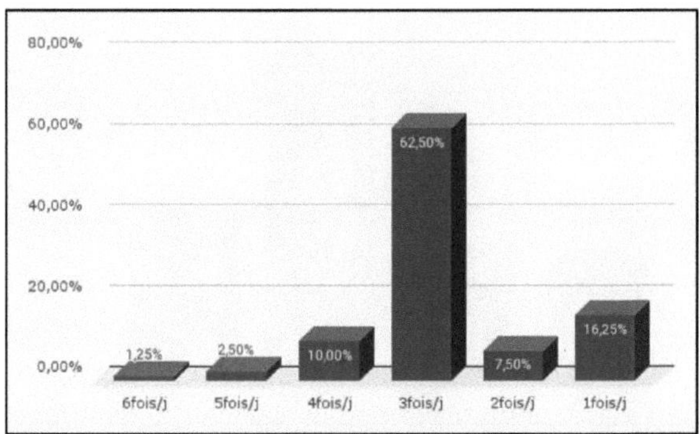

Figure 33: Distribution of nurses by frequency of disinfecting workplaces

Most respondents (62.5%) disinfect their workplaces 3 times a day while a minority of 1% disinfect them 6 times a day.

1.5. Distribution of nurses according to knowledge of universal precautions for Blood Exposure Accidents (BEA) :

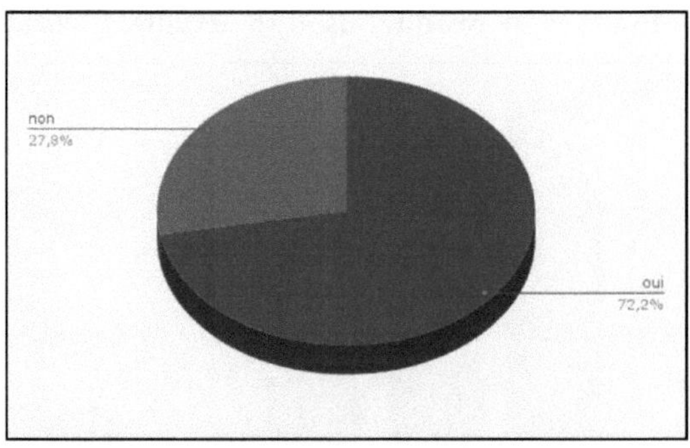

Figure 34: Distribution of nurses according to knowledge of Universal precautions for Blood Exposure Accidents (BSE) According to our results, 72% of those questioned were aware of the universal precautions for BSE...

1.6. Distribution of nurses according to knowledge of measures forming part of universal precautions for AES :

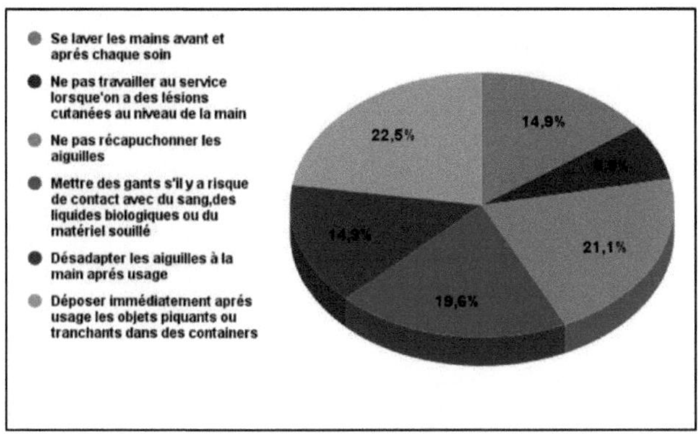

Figure 35: Distribution of nurses according to knowledge of measures forming part of universal precautions for AES :

We find that 22.5% of the population thought that disposing of sharps in containers immediately after use was a universal precaution for AES. Whereas 21% thought that not recapping needles was a universal precaution for AES. 19% chose the option: wear gloves if there is a risk of contact with the skin. blood, biological products or soiled materials. 30% of respondents felt that washing their hands before and after each treatment and removing needles from their hands after use are among the universal precautions for AES.Only 6.9% believed that not working on the ward when you have skin lesions on your hand. 19% chose the suggestion: wear gloves if there is a risk of contact with blood, biological products or soiled materials. 30% of respondents indicated that washing their hands before and after each treatment and removing needles from their hands after use are among the universal precautions for AES. Only 6.9% thought that not working in the department when you have skin lesions on the hand

1.7. Distribution of nurses according to suggestions for improving knowledge of HAIs and their prevention :

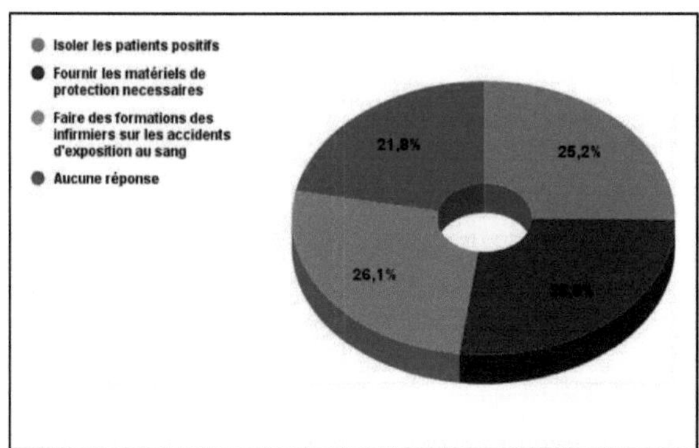

Figure 36: Distribution of nurses according to suggestions for improving knowledge of HAIs and their prevention :

27% of respondents stressed the importance of providing the necessary protection, and training nurses in the prevention of SEA and 25 suggested isolating positive patients.

1.8. Distribution of nurses according to knowledge of treatment against hepatitis C :

A. Distribution of nurses according to availability of treatment against hepatitis C :

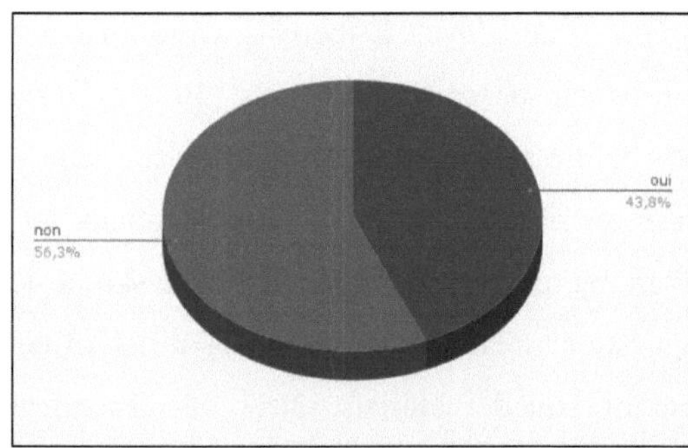

Figure 37: Distribution of nurses by availability of medical treatment for hepatitis C

56.3% of respondents replied that there was no medical treatment against hepatitis C.

1.9. Distribution of nurses according to knowledge of medical treatment for hepatitis C :

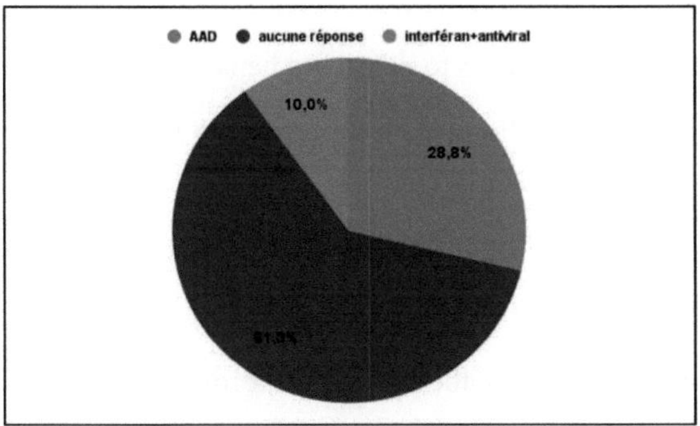

Figure 38: Distribution of nurses according to knowledge of medical treatment for hepatitis C

• The majority of the population (61.3) did not answer this question.

• 29% of nurses indicated that direct-acting antivirals (DAAs) represent the medical treatment for hepatitis C.

1.10. Distribution of nurses according to availability of hepatitis C vaccine :

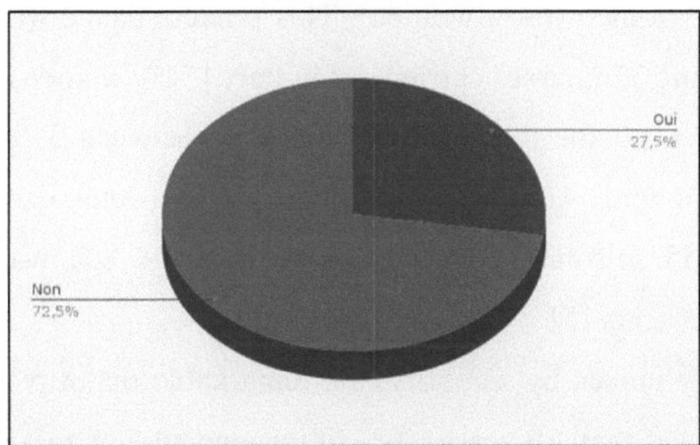

Figure 39: Distribution of nurses by availability of hepatitis C vaccine

According to 72% of staff questioned, there is no effective vaccine against hepatitis C.

DISCUSSION

The Global Health Strategy aims to eliminate hepatitis as a major threat to public health by 2030. The hepatitis C virus (HCV) can be difficult to detect, as infection can remain asymptomatic for decades. This highlights the importance of increasing knowledge among healthcare providers in order to achieve viral hepatitis targets [3].

Our study attempted to assess the current state of knowledge of nurses at the University Hospital of Gabès about HCV infection, transmission, prevention and treatment, and to identify gaps and shortcomings with a view to devising a public health action plan to correct and improve knowledge and management.

I. Population identification :

The results of our study show that nurses are divided into 12 departments. During the study period, 80 nurses were included. The sex ratio was 0.56, with a predominance of women (64% women). This predominance was also observed in a study including 326 nurses carried out in Italy (54% women) [4].

In our study, 58% of the respondents were aged between 31 and 50, with an average age of 33, while 41% were aged under 30. In a study carried out in 2003 and including 935 self-employed nurses, the average age was 44.6 with an average age of 33 years [5].

When we classify nurses by seniority, the remarkable majority have been with the company for less than 10 years (80% of respondents), which is This is in line with the results of a survey carried out in Morocco, where almost half the population qualified for less than 10 years [6].Our questionnaire was distributed to 12 wards at the University Hospital of Gabès, which appeared to us to be wards that could receive and treat patients with HCV. While a study carried out in Italy was limited to haemodialysis units because of the increased risk of transmission of this infection in these services[4].

II. Assessment of general knowledge about hepatitis C:

1. Definition:

According to the WHO, "Hepatitis C is an inflammation of the liver caused by the hepatitis C virus. The manifestations of hepatitis C can be acute, chronic and benign or serious and irreversible, such as cirrhosis and cancer. Acute HCV infections are usually asymptomatic and most do not lead to life-threatening illness. Around 30% (15% to 45%) of those infected spontaneously eliminate the virus within six months of infection without any treatment. For the remaining 70% (55% to 85%) of infected people, the infection will progress to the chronic form of the disease. Among these chronic patients, the risk of cirrhosis is 15% to 30% over a 20-year period". [7].

2. The officer in charge :

According to wikipedia The hepatitis C virus (HCV) is a small RNA virus approximately 60 nanometres in diameter, enveloped i n an icosahedral protein capsid. Its genome is a single-stranded linear RNA of positive polarity. There are six major genotypes of hepatitis C virus, indicated by a number [8].

In our study, almost the entire population knew that the agent responsible for of hepatitis C is a virus.

3. Modes of transmission :

❖**Transmission by blood can occur :**

•Following a blood exposure accident (BEA): after occupational exposure to HCV through needlesticks, the transmission rate is estimated at around 1 to 3%. The transmission rate is around 10 times lower after exposure to mucous membranes or injured skin.

•By sharing injection equipment (syringe, spoon, filter, water) among IV drug users. This is the main mode of transmission of HCV. Drug use by nasal route (sharing straws) or by smoked route (sharing crack pipes) is also a risk factor for HCV transmission.

· During blood transfusions, when transfusion safety measures are not applied

· When tattooing or piercing with non-sterile equipment;

❖ **Sexual transmission**

• is extremely low, can occur:

• when the penis penetrates the vagina or anus. The risk of sexual transmission is rarer, but it increases during anal sex, which can cause lesions or injuries, such as inserting fingers or a fist into the anus in the presence of blood.

❖ **Maternal-foetal transmission**: only occurs when the mother is viremic.

It follows from the above that the population at risk of hepatitis C is represented by :

► **Exhibiting activities**

Healthcare workers, laboratory staff who handle blood samples, people likely to come into contact with sharp objects contaminated with blood.

► **Land at increased risk of acquisition**

Injecting drug users, haemodialysis patients.

► **Terrain at increased risk of severe disease**

Alcoholism; co-infections with HBV or HIV, which increase the risk of developing cirrhosis. Chronic HBsAg carriage may favour the development of acute fulminant hepatitis C.

► **Pregnancy**

-Pregnant women: no particularities.

-Unborn child: low risk of contamination [9].

In our study, we found that half of the staff questioned knew that the hepatitis c virus is transmitted mainly by blood, while the other modes of transmission (sexual and maternal-foetal) were mentioned less frequently.

In a cross-sectional survey of nurses in the Calabria region (Italy), 49.8% correctly identified all the routes of HCV transmission; Most of the nurses had a good knowledge of some of the ways to transmissions among the following: receiving a blood transfusion from an infected donor (93.9%), having sex with an HCV-positive partner (91.4%) and exchanging needles when injecting drugs (90.7%),11.5% believed that HCV could be transmitted by a kissing and 19.2% did not mention tattooing as a route of hepatitis C transmission [4].

4. Means of transmission of hepatitis C :

Hepatitis c is transmitted in healthcare settings by various means:
• The risk concerns healthcare workers or any other person in the event of a needle stick or a cut with a sharp object soiled with the blood of an HCV-infected person.
• There is also a low risk if the blood of an HCV-infected person is spilt on a wound, injured skin or mucous membrane (as mentioned by 18% of respondents).

• The average risk of transmission following percutaneous exposure to the blood of a infected patient is between 0.5 and 3% [10].

• These means of transmission were mentioned by our population, with a predominance of needlestick injuries (43.42%). Some also mentioned spraying blood on injured skin or mucous membranes (49.34%) as a risk factor for transmission of the virus.
• However, these means of transmission were mentioned with high percentages by Moroccan nurses in a similar study: contact with blood on injured skin (91.7%), needlesticks (83.5%), blood spray on mucous membranes (82.7%), sexual contact (44.1%) and blood spray on healthy skin (7.5%) [6].

II. Complications of hepatitis C :

1. Cirrhosis :

Cirrhosis occurs in 20% of cases, when the liver presents a series of diffuse and irreversible lesions. Fibrosis destroys the structure of the liver and creates abnormal nodules, with portal hypertension and hepatocellular insufficiency that can lead to a number of complications such as haemorrhage from ruptured oesophageal varices, ascites, jaundice or encephalopathy. In addition, cirrhotic livers are favourable sites for the development of cancer because they contain genetic alterations. These complications occur with a frequency of 15-20% over 4 years in patients with cirrhosis.

2. Hepatocellular carcinoma

Hepatocellular carcinoma (HCC) is the most common primary liver cancer. In the majority of cases, it occurs in a liver damaged by chronic disease, most often at the stage of cirrhosis at the time of diagnosis. Cirrhosis due to chronic hepatitis is the leading cause of hepatocellular carcinoma in Europe and the second in France. HCC is one of the cancers with the highest mortality rate, around 95% at 5 years.

3. Extra-hepatic manifestations :

•Chronic hepatitis C leads to a number of extra-hepatic symptoms:
•Mixed cryoglobulinemias, which cause cryoglobulinemic vasculitides. Deposits of immune complexes accumulate in the small vessels (arterioles, venules and capillaries) and progressively reduce their calibre, causing a lack of irrigation to the tissues and even tissue necrosis. As a result, there may be several 18 clinical manifestations, including skin, kidney, rheumatological, neurological, cardiac, salivary and respiratory disorders.
•. In dermatology: porphyria cutanea tarda, pruritus and lichen planus, the

mechanisms of which are still poorly understood.

•Certain thyroid disorders, dry syndrome, porphyria cutanea tarda, non-Hodgkin's lymphoma. However, the causal link has not been clearly established.

•Other manifestations such as diabetes, insulin resistance, certain cardiovascular pathologies and cognitive disorders are more frequently observed in patients with chronic hepatitis C. However, the mechanisms involved are diverse and poorly documented [11].

•In this context, half of our patients cited cirrhosis as the main complication of hepatitis C, and extra-hepatic manifestations were not mentioned.

•In the same context, the results of a study carried out in France showed that 46% believe that HC constantly progresses to cirrhosis and in 50% of cases to HCC [5].

4. Means of prevention :

Reduction in the incidence of work-related HCV infections depends on three factors:

■a reduction in risk, in particular by avoiding high-risk gestures (ban on recapping manoeuvres, use of containers, etc.). for used needles and safe single-use equipment);

■compliance with recommendations in the event of an accident involving exposure to blood (cleaning the wound, reporting, monitoring) ;

■early treatment of acute viral hepatitis C to limit the risk of transition to chronicity. In fact, compliance with the recommendations appears to be a key factor, since the monitoring of blood exposure accidents involving an HCV-positive "source patient" carried out over several years in the hospitals of the Assistance Publique de Paris and the Hospices Civils de Marseille shows a seroconversion rate of 0% [12].

In our study, respondents emphasised vaccination and sterilisation of equipment as the main means of preventing hepatitis C.

IV. Hepatitis C prevention practices in care environment :

1. Hand washing and disinfection

The importance of hand washing in preventing the transmission of infectious agents has been known for many years, but all too often it is not applied sufficiently. Various reasons are given for this: intolerance to soaps, lack of time, lack of equipment at water points _ This observation has prompted the promotion of new hand hygiene techniques, such as hand disinfection with a hydroalcoholic product. This technique of rubbing hands with a product with a high alcohol content (hydroalcoholic solution or gel) is recognised as effective. It enables rapid hand hygiene, even when there is no equipped water point close to the point of care, such as at the patient's home or in an emergency situation. Its use has been recommended by the Comité Technique des Infections Nosocomiales since December 2001. The following terminology and recommendations are largely based on those issued by the French Hospital Hygiene Society in 2002. The products chosen must comply with clearly defined standards. It is usual to distinguish between several types of hand washing or disinfection, each with its own effectiveness, technique and indications. The choice of technique will depend on how dirty the hands are, the level of infectious risk associated with the procedure being or having been carried out, and the equipment available at the point of care:

•**Simple hand washing:** Operation designed to remove dirt and reduce transient flora by mechanical action, using soap and water.

•**Hygienic hand washing and hygienic hand treatment by friction:** Operation designed to eliminate or reduce transient flora, by washing or friction using a disinfectant product.

•**Surgical hand disinfection by washing:** Operation designed to eliminate transient flora and reduce resident flora over a prolonged period, by surgical washing or surgical disinfection by friction using a disinfectant product or a combination of simple washing and surgical friction [13].

•In this context, the majority of nurses interviewed in our study respect hand washing, whereas in Morocco hand disinfection with soap was practised regularly by only 63% of subjects, compared with 6 8 in France [6].

2. Wearing gloves:

Wearing gloves does not replace hand washing or disinfection. They protect carers and patients by preventing cross-transmission. Gloves should be worn on hands with short fingernails and no rings or other jewellery.

One pair of gloves = one procedure = one patient Caution when "interrupting care!

1.2. Single-use non-sterile gloves :

They are used to prevent cross-transmission by manu portage and operator protection whenever there is a risk of contact with :

– Blood or any other biological product

– Injured skin or mucous membranes

– Soiled linen or equipment,

• during care, whenever the carer presents a skin lesion at the level of the skin. hands.

By limiting the amount of dirt on the hands, they make it easier to wash or disinfect them when they are removed. They protect the operator from the risk of contact with blood or a biological product. Examples: blood sampling, insertion and removal of a peripheral venous line, removal of a soiled dressing, wound cleansing, emptying a urinary catheter, subcutaneous, intramuscular or intravenous injections, examination of mucous membranes, dental care, waste handling

2.2. Single-use sterile gloves

They will be used for :

• all procedures requiring a high level of asepsis,

• any handling of sterile products and materials.

Examples: suturing, inserting a urinary catheter, handling an implantable chamber, inserting an IUD, treating a wound without sterile forceps, invasive dental care. They are sold sterile in individual packaging.

3. Wearing a smock:

Wearing a single-use protective gown is recommended:

• during care that may expose the carer's clothing to splashes of blood or biological fluids ("Standard" precautions)
• during treatment of a patient requiring contact precautions. They must be reserved for care given to a single patient.

4. Wearing a mask :

A distinction is made between :

- **medical masks** (care masks, surgical masks) are designed to prevent droplets of saliva or respiratory secretions from being projected when exhalation from the carer to the patient or from a contagious patient to those around him. Certain models, which include an impermeable layer and sometimes a visor, can also protect the carer against liquid splashes from the patient during care or surgery; these are known as anti-splash masks. Under no circumstances can they protect the wearer from inhaling infectious particles. These masks must comply with European Directive 93/42/EEC on medical devices (class I medical devices).

- **disposable respiratory protection masks** consist of a half-mask covering the mouth and nose. They are designed to protect the wearer against inhalation of dust and/or aerosols contaminated with airborne infectious agents. There are three classes of effectiveness: FFP1, FFP2, FFP3. The effectiveness of the mask is limited in time. The effectiveness of a mask also depends in part on how well it fits on the face. It is advisable to consult the instructions for use supplied by the manufacturers. Once the mask is in place, handling should be avoided, as this encourages contamination of the hands and deterioration of the mask. Hands should be washed after removal.

In town, wearing a mask is recommended for :

- Patient protection

When performing technical procedures requiring a high level of asepsis (e.g. implantable chamber dressings, interventional radiology procedures, fibroscopy procedures, etc.), a care or surgical mask should be worn by the carer. A carer with a respiratory infection should refrain from providing any care to an immunocompromised patient, or alternatively should provide such care wearing a surgical mask.

- Protecting healthcare professionals

During treatment involving a risk of splashing blood or biological fluids (dental care, fibroscopy, chiropody, etc.), an anti-splash mask must be worn by the healthcare professional. In this case, the wearing of goggles A protective goggle or face mask is also recommended. (When caring for patients with an infection requiring special precautions, essentially where there is a risk of transmission by the "airborne" route (A) or by the "droplet" route (G), with a risk of aerosolisation, a respiratory protection mask should be worn by the healthcare professional [13].

In the literature, a study carried out in Morocco showed that the systematic use of protective equipment against AES was not observed by the majority of staff: 35.2% did not systematically wear a gown and 75.6% and 72.3% did not systematically wear gloves and a bib during treatment respectively [6].

V. Evaluation of attitudes and practices towards risk of hepatitis C :

1. Contaminating products :

1.1. Cloths stained with blood:

Clean and dirty linen are among the main vectors of infection: they are ideal breeding grounds for germs,

2.1. Blood and biological products containing blood :

Blood: bleeding, menstrual blood, Lochies (during childbirth). In our study, soiled cloths were the contaminating materials handled the most, followed (38%) by blood-contaminated puncture fluids (27%) and contaminated genital swab waste (22%). Biopsy products containing blood were cited by only 13% of participants.

•Any biological product contaminated with the blood of a patient carrying hepatitis risks transmitting the virus to the carer in the event of an accident involving a prick or the spraying of blood onto a carer's mucous membrane or injured skin.

In a similar study carried out in Morocco, the contaminants most frequently handled were blood (91.3%) followed by soiled linen (67.4%).%) , waste (51.5%), puncture fluid (45.9%) , sputum (26.3%) %), genital samples (10%) and biopsy material (9.3%).%)[6].

2. Contaminating materials :

Any medical equipment that has come into contact with the blood of a patient carrying the HCV virus is considered to be contaminated and may be a means of transmitting hepatitis C to healthcare workers.

Exposure to the blood or biological fluids of viral serology-positive patients through contaminating medical equipment can lead to :

• **Significant risk in the** event of a deep wound or with a hollow needle for venous or arterial sampling containing blood or with a catheter used.

• **Intermediate risk** if it involves a needle previously used for subcutaneous or intramuscular injection, a solid needle such as a suture needle or a scalpel needle.

• **The risk is low in the** case of needlestick injuries involving discarded needles, which either contain no blood or have coagulated blood [14].

In this context, our nurses mentioned that hollow needles were the main contaminating material (34.81%), while only 1/4 handled scalpels. In a similar Moroccan study, the risk materials handled by staff were, in decreasing order of frequency, hollow needles (77.9%), scalpels (64.4%), interannuals (52.4%), epicranials (45.4%), catheters (31.1%) and solid needles (33.5%).%) [6].

3. Hand disinfection products :

Hand hygiene and disinfection: which products to choose?

For years, the health authorities have been pointing out that bacteria, germs and viruses are easily transmitted via the hands and fingernails. Disinfecting hands properly kills micro-organisms on the skin, thereby avoiding any risk of transmission. There's a whole range of biocidal products (hydroalcoholic gel, foams, soaps, etc.) to make life easier if traditional hand washing isn't possible. It's true that some pathogens can survive washing with ordinary soap and water, but afterwards they are enveloped in soap molecules and washed away by the rinse water.

✓ Antibacterial soaps:

Antibacterial soaps are generally considered to be excessive in most cases.

Hospitals are an exception to this rule because of the particular situations they encounter (before invasive procedures, when caring for immunocompromised patients, in intensive care areas, in intensive care nurseries, etc.).Antibacterial agents should be chosen carefully according to their characteristics and active ingredients, and when persistent antibacterial or antimicrobial action on the hands is desired.

✓ **Disinfectants:**

Where there is no access to soap and water, a hand sanitiser or antiseptic product (without water) can b e used.Some of these products contain ethyl alcohol combined with emollients (to soften the skin) and other agents. They are often presented in the form of :

gel, wipes or wet towels

To be effective, alcohol-based hand sanitisers should contain at least 60% alcohol. These products do not eliminate all types of pathogens.

Hand sanitisers can also give off an odour that some users find unpleasant.

To use a hand disinfectant correctly, you need to :

• Apply the amount recommended by the manufacturer to the palm of the hand.
• Rubbing hands.

• Spread the product over the whole hand and rub until the hands are dry.

• Use enough product to coat hands and fingers completely.

Alcohol-based hand sanitisers are the method of choice for healthcare providers when hands are not visibly dirty. These products can also be used by ambulance technicians, home care assistants and other mobile workers in the absence of a w a s h r o o m . hand-washing facilities. These alcohol-based disinfectants(at least 60%) are also recommended for the general public in the event of a pandemic.

However, these agents are not effective when hands are heavily contaminated with dirt, blood or other organic matter.Hand washing with soap and water is recommended when hands are visibly dirty. [15].In this context, the majority of nurses taking part in our survey disinfect their hands with soap or bleach.In a similar study carried out in Morocco, soap or bleach were not used regularly to disinfect hands by just 63% of people. Alcohol at 70° and other antiseptics (iodine derivatives, organomercurials, hexamidine, quaternary ammoniums) were used systematically by only 45% of carers. [6].

4. Disinfection of medical equipment :

The disinfection procedure must be adapted to the risk involved. Effective disinfection involves assessing the risk of infection. The nature of the procedure and the fragility of the patient are the two components of this assessment. The treatment required is therefore adapted according to the level of risk and the medical equipment used. Instruments coming into contact with a mucous membrane or injured skin (gastroscope, colonoscope, etc.) are classified as semi-critical with a medium risk of infection. Disinfection will be of intermediate level. Instruments in contact with intact patient skin or without direct contact are considered non-critical. As the risk of contamination is low, disinfection will be low level. The level of requirement for equipment and treatment must also take into account the level of asepsis in the environment (operating theatre, treatment room, room).

Steps and procedures for effective disinfection :

The medical equipment will undergo various stages which will determine the effectiveness of the disinfection.

✓ Pre-treatment

This step is necessary to facilitate cleaning, reduce the level of contamination and protect staff and the environment. Medical instruments must be immersed in a soaking tank with a detergent that may be bactericidal. Cleaning The cleaning protocol removes dirt. Effective cleaning reduces the microbial load that could inactivate the product during disinfection. Cleaning combines four actions: mechanical (brushing), chemical (detergent), immersion time and temperature. Cleaning can be done manually or using a suitable washing machine such as an ultrasonic tank.

✓ Disinfection

It destroys or inactivates micro-organisms. There are two disinfection methods. The chemical method involves immersing medical instruments in a disinfectant solution or using specific equipment. Disinfectants are chosen according to the level of disinfection required (bactericide, fungicide, virucide, mycobactericide or sporicide). The thermal or chemical-thermal method is most often carried out using specific equipment: steam disinfectors, washing and disinfecting machines, bedpan washers. It is essential to rinse the equipment thoroughly with tap water (possibly fitted with a filter) between each of the above stages [15].

In our study, most of the population studied often disinfected equipment with heat, and 47% of respondents disinfected equipment with soap or bleach. In a study carried out in Moroccan hospitals, equipment was disinfected using bleach at 12°C diluted 1:10 and soap in 57.7% of cases, alcohol at 70°C in 8.6%, iodine derivatives in 11.4% and heat (Poupinel) in 6.4% of cases [16].

5. Products and frequency of disinfection of treatment areas :

It is recommended that floors, furniture surfaces and equipment be cleaned daily and immediately in the event of soiling (professional agreement). It is recommended that maintenance procedures are written down and made available in the form of a protocol, specifying the equipment required, the tasks to be performed, their allocation and the frequency with which they should be carried out (professional agreement).Damp dusting (wet sweeping) is the essential preliminary step to floor cleaning. For surfaces other than floors, damp wiping with a detergent or detergent-disinfectant is generally the only step.Simple floor cleaning, i.e. damp dusting followed by the use of a commercial detergent, is recommended for all areas of the surgery (professional agreement). For surfaces other than floors, wet wiping is recommended (professional agreement):

•with a detergent in the reception and secretarial areas, the waiting room and the filing room

•with a detergent-disinfectant1 in the examination and treatment room, the lingerie, sanitary facilities, cleaning room, waste storage room, medical device processing area, medical device packaging area prior to sterilisation, sterilisation area and sterile equipment and drug storage area.

We recommend cleaning and disinfecting the table. after examining a patient. Clean and then disinfect surfaces soiled by splashes of blood or any other product of human origin with Bleach® with 2.6% chlorine freshly diluted to 1/10° (or any other appropriate disinfectant) [17].

In our study, according to the majority of the population (60%), surfanios is the main product used for disinfecting workplaces 3 times a day (according to antiseptic (62%). In a Moroccan study, disinfection of work premises was only carried out consistently in 73.1% of cases, with a frequency of once a day (17%), three times a week (28.4%) and once a month (27.7%) [6].

6. AES precautions :

General hygiene precautions must be applied when there is a risk of SEA:

✓ Comply with current recommendations on washing and disinfecting hands, in particular washing immediately in the event of contact with

potentially contaminating biological fluids.

✓ Wear gloves:

• if there is a risk of contact with blood or any other product of human origin, with the mucous membranes or injured skin of a patient, particularly during treatment involving the risk of needlestick injuries and when handling tubes or bottles of biological samples, soiled linen and equipment;

• and systematically in the event of skin lesions on the hands.

Changing them between two patients, two activities.

Certain situations may require additional precautions: wearing two pairs of gloves, particularly for operators in operating theatres, and wearing cut-resistant under-gloves for particularly high-risk procedures, especially in anatomical pathology.

✓ When there is a risk of blood or potentially contaminating biological products being sprayed, wear appropriate clothing (anti-spray surgical mask with goggles or face shield),

overblouse).

✓ Preferably use single-use equipment.

✓ Use the medical safety devices provided.

✓ Respect good practice when handling instruments soiled sharps :

• never recap the needles;

• do not remove needles from syringes or vacuum sampling systems by hand;

• dispose of needles and other sharp instruments immediately, without handling them, in a suitable container (in accordance with the amended Order of 24 November 2003), as close as possible to the treatment area, with an easily accessible opening and not exceeding the maximum filling level;

• if reusable equipment is used, when it is soiled, the handle with care and ensure prompt and appropriate treatment.

✓ Biological samples, linen and instruments soiled with

Blood or biological products must be transported, including within the establishment, in appropriate sealed packaging, then treated or disposed of if necessary through defined channels [18]. This data is consistent with that provided by our study, since most of these precautions are mentioned by the respondents.

7. Measures to improve knowledge about HAIs and their prevention :

7.1. Vaccination status

Vaccination against hepatitis B is compulsory for all healthcare professionals, including self-employed workers. To ensure that your vaccinations are up to date, please refer to the vaccination calendar.

7.2. Compliance with general hygiene precautions

Known as "Standard Precautions", they are set out in circular no. 98/249 of 20 April 1998 on preventing the transmission of infectious agents carried by blood or biological fluids during healthcare.

7.3. Information and training for professionals

Inform and train staff on :

• the risk of HAI and the preventive measures to be applied ;

• the importance of vaccination ; what to do in the event of an SEA

WHAT TO DO IN THE EVENT OF AN ACCIDENT

EXPOSING TO BLOOD

EMERGENCY FIRST AID

In the event of a sting or wound :

Do not bleed

• Immediately cleanse the affected skin area with soap and water, then rinse

• Antisepsis with a chlorine derivative (Dakin or bleach with 2.6% active chlorine diluted 1:5) or a povidone-iodine dermal solution or, failing that, 70° alcohol (at least 5 minutes).

► In the event of direct contact of the biological fluid with injured skin :

• The same protocols for cleaning and antisepsis of the affected area as for previously

► In case of splashing on mucous membranes and eyes :

• Rinse w i t h plenty of water or saline solution (at least 5 minutes).

❖SEEK MEDICAL ADVICE QUICKLY: CONTACT A REFERRING DOCTOR

► Who assesses the risk of infection :

Investigation of the serological status of the source person :

√ HIV status :

-If the source person is HIV-negative, there is no need for further monitoring, unless there is a risk of ongoing primary infection in the source person: if in doubt, carry out a viral load test.

–If the source subject's HIV status is not known and is available, HIV serology should be carried out with the subject's consent (except in cases where consent cannot be expressed), if possible. with a rapid test (TROD) in order to start an EIPT as quickly as possible in the exposed person.

–In the case of HIV infection, it is essential to have the result of the last HIV plasma viral load, as well as the nature of previous and current antiretroviral treatments, and their virological efficacy.

If the HIV-infected source patient has been on antiretroviral treatment with an undetectable viral load for more than six months, the risk of transmission via the bloodstream is considered to be zero.

A viral load should be offered as a matter of urgency to source patients if they are accessible and if no recent results are available (less than six months) or if there is any doubt about compliance with treatment. It is therefore legitimate to initiate an EBCT while waiting for this information.

✓ **but also the HCV** and possibly **HBV status** if the victim is not not immune.

► **Who informs you of the measures to be taken:**

You may be offered prophylaxis (**post-exposure treatment**, specific anti-HBV immunoglobulins >+/- vaccination). You will be given prior information about the effects of this treatment and how it will be carried out. Your consent is required. Treatment must be started within hours of the accident.

Set up **medical and serological monitoring** for hepatitis B and C.

In the event of exposure to HIV, serological monitoring is essential for **compensation** in the event of seroconversion.

❖ **REPORT THE ACCIDENT**

As the practical arrangements vary from one establishment to another and from one social security scheme to another, you should obtain information from your occupational physician, manager or personnel office [19].

In our study :

o 26.9% of respondents stressed the importance of providing the necessary protective equipment and training nurses in AES, 25% suggested isolating positive patients and 21% did not answer this question.

Whereas in a Moroccan study carried out to assess knowledge of AES, staff wanted training and information courses on AES (51.3%), correct and well-conducted vaccination (47.3%), better availability of means of protection (32.2%), better hygiene in workplaces (36.2%), the introduction of an occupational health service in hospitals with reinforced medical surveillance of exposed individuals (28.5%), compulsory reporting of HAIs (28.5%) and proper waste management (12.3%) [6].

■**Medical treatment of hepatitis C :**

At present, we have treatments that can be divided into

three families:

x Treatment with immunomodulating agents

x Treatment with direct-acting antivirals (DAAs)

x Treatment with host-directed antivirals.

■**Immunomodulating agents**

► **Interferons**

Interferons are glycoproteins belonging to the cytokine family. endogenous. They are produced by the body in response to various stimuli, particularly viral infections. They play a role in regulating resistance to viral infections and activating the innate or adaptive immune response. IFNDs are used in the treatment of chronic HCV infection.These molecules have antiviral, antiproliferative, antifibrosing and immunomodulatory properties. Finally, IFN has anti-inflammatory and anti-fibrosing properties.

► **Ribavirin :**

Ribavirin is a nucleoside guanosine analogue that has shown antiviral activity against HCV. Several mechanisms of action are involved. Firstly, ribavirin has the ability to inhibit RNA capping activity and that of viral RNA polymerase. The use of ribavirin alone in the treatment of HCV gives limited and transient results, and is best used in combination with IFN, whose antiviral effect it potentiates.

■**Direct-acting antivirals :**

DAAs include several molecules, namely NS3-4A protease inhibitors, nucleotide and non-nucleotide inhibitors of NS5B polymerase and NS5A complex inhibitors.

► **NS3-4A protease inhibitors:**

NS3-4A protease inhibitors were the first direct-acting antivirals to be introduced as part of HCV control strategies. These molecules have the ability to bind covalently but reversibly to the Serine (Ser169) of the NS3 protease active site. This binding leads to inhibition of the NS3/4A protease, thereby preventing the replication and production of viral particles.

► **Nucleoside inhibitors of NS5B polymerase**

The basic principle is the use of a nucleotide analogue that competes with the natural substrate to bind to the active site of the RNA-dependent RNA polymerase. This analogue also has a chain-terminating effect after incorporation into the newly synthesised RNA, thereby inhibiting viral replication.

► **Non-nucleoside inhibitors of NS5B polymerase** These molecules inhibit enzymatic activity by binding to one of the four allosteric sites on the surface of the enzyme, leading to an alteration in the conformation of the enzyme. polymerase, blocking its catalytic function and therefore RNA replication

► **NS5A complex inhibitors**

They inhibit both viral RNA replication and virion assembly. These properties are linked to their dual action on the NS5A protein: interaction with its N-terminal region, leading to the formation of structural distortions, and blockage of its hyperphosphorylation, which is necessary for it to function properly.

■ **Host-directed antivirals**

Numerous studies have identified the host molecules that play a crucial role in virion entry or replication. These new targets could therefore be considered in the treatment of hepatitis C.These include microRNA-122, viral coreceptors and cyclophilins. Unfortunately, treatments to inhibit these molecules are still under study. genotypes 2 and 3. The high level of HCV viral replication is thought to be one of the main causes of failure [20]. Most of our staff are not familiar with the treatment of CCH and so did not answer this question. In a Canadian study carried out in 2017, only 21% of participating nurses did not know about direct-acting antiviral treatments for HCV [21].

■ Is there a vaccine available against hepatitis C?

There is currently no preventive vaccine against hepatitis C, but some laboratories are working on "therapeutic vaccines" designed to treat patients already suffering from the disease.The new product has been successfully tested on mice and monkeys, but not yet on humans. The trials showed that the vaccine triggered a strong response from certain so-called neutralising antibodies, which fought off various variants of the hepatitis C virus, the researchers reported on Wednesday."For a preventive vaccine, neutralising antibodies are absolutely essential, and they would also be a great advantage for a therapeutic product", emphasised David Klatzmann, one of the members of the team [22].In our study, more than half the population correctly believe that there is no vaccine for hepatitis C, while 44% falsely believe that there i s an effective vaccine against the disease.

■ Study limits :

Our results give us an idea of the knowledge of nurses working at the University Hospital of Gabès about chronic hepatitis C. However, some limitations are highlighted.Bearing in mind that the study involved nurses from the hospital's 12 departments the interpretation and generalisation of the results to all the universities in Gabès. Tunisian nurses must be carefully discussed since our study was not addressed to all nurses working in hospitals. Another limitation of our study is the small size of our sample, and the unequal distribution of men and women in this study population. The data in our study was filled in by the participants themselves, and this may represent a bias that is common in this type of study. However, this bias was minimised by the anonymous and confidential nature of our study.

RECOMMENDATIONS

It is strongly recommended that a wide range of training courses be developed for nurses on the subject of infections and hygiene, with the aim of increasing their knowledge in this area.More funding is needed to provide the medical equipment needed to treat infections such as hepatitis C, and to prevent HAI in healthcare settings and the transmission of these diseases to healthcare workers. It is also proposed to focus these types of studies to improve the state of nursing knowledge about hepatitis C and to highlight this development.

CONCLUSION

Infection with the hepatitis C virus (HCV) is considered to be a major public health problem worldwide, due to its frequency and seriousness, with a high risk of progression to cirrhosis.The WHO estimated that around 3% of the general population was infected with this disease.virus [2].However, this prevalence varies between three geographical zones: high prevalence of between 1.5% and 6%, medium prevalence of 1% and low prevalence of less than 0.5%. Tunisia is a low-endemic country for hepatitis C, with a prevalence of no more than 1% in the general population. The main routes of HCV infection are drug use and parenteral administration for diagnostic or therapeutic purposes. In the majority of cases, the disease is completely asymptomatic, and is discovered by chance in the presence of elevated transaminases, during a blood donation, or when suffering from fatigue, or during screening; extra-hepatic manifestations can sometimes be revealing. In recent years, great progress has been made in the treatment of HCV, and the infection is now curable. Previous treatment programmes were based on PEG-Interferon and ribavirin, which required longer periods of treatment and had more side effects. The new interferon-free direct-acting antiviral (DAA) treatments have been shown to be highly effective, with fewer side effects, and there is currently no vaccine against hepatitis C [23]. The prevalence of chronic hepatitis C and the recognised developments in care and treatment make it necessary to improve nurses' knowledge of this infectious disease, as they are among the carers most confronted with this health problem. This context led us to carry out a descriptive study on a sample of 80 nurses practising in 12 departments at the University Hospital of Gabès with the aim of evaluating the state of nursing knowledge about hepatitis C.Our results show that our population is sometimes unaware of certain details that require awareness-raising and training to improve knowledge of this disease.

.

BIBLIOGRAPHY

(1) Hepatitis C - symptoms, causes, treatment and prevention-VIDAL. (n.d.). Accessed 9 June 2023, at https://www.vidal.fr/maladies/estomac-intestins/hepatite-c.html

(2) Tunisian Consensus Meeting (rns.tn)

(3) Canada, Public Health A. (2018, January 4). Health care providers' knowledge of hepatitis C [Education and awareness]. https://www.canada.ca/fr/sante-publique/services/rapports-publications/releve-maladies- transmissibles-canada-rmtc/numero-mensuel/2018-44/numero-7-8-5-july-2018/article- 2-knowledge-hepatitis-c-health-care-providers.html

(4) Healthcare workers and prevention of hepatitis C virus transmission: exploring knowledge, attitudes and evidence-based practices in hemodialysis units in Italy I BMC Infectious Diseases I Text .) Retrieved June 9, 2023, fromHealthcare workers and prevention of hepatitis C virus transmission: exploring knowledge, attitudes and evidence-based practices in hemodialysis units in Italy | BMC Infectious Diseases | Full Text (biomedcentral.com)

(5) CHRONIC HEPATITIS C: NURSING KNOWLEDGE AND PRACTICE LIBERALS (survey and training of the vhc 91-77 network) (2003, October 1). Abstracts of ANGH congresses. Accessed 9 June 2023 at https://angh.net/abstracts/hepatite- chronique-c-connaissances-et-pratique-des-infirmiers-liberauxenquete-et-formation-du- reseau-vhc-91-77/

(6) Evaluation of knowledge, attitudes and practices concerning viral hepatitis B and C in health care settings in Morocco . Retrieved June 9, 2023, from Évaluation des connaissances, attitudes et pratiques sur les hépatites virales B et C en milieu de soins au Maroc | Cairn.info

(7) Key facts about hepatitis C. (n.d.). Accessed 9 June 2023, at https://www.who.int/fr/news-room/fact-sheets/detail/hepatitis-c

(8) Hepatitis C - Wikipedia. (n.d.). Retrieved June 9, 2023, from

https://fr.m.wikipedia.org/wiki/H%C3%A9patite_C?fbclid=IwAR1blgaAPmtVP6 W8NgQ FUEQUfZX-xeU210Xxp-ZTxx57hkg872BslcrSDQk

(9) Modes of transmission of viral hepatitis - devsante.org. (n.d.). Accessed 9 June 2023, at address https://devsante.org/articles/modes-de-transmission-des-hepatites-virales/

(10) Mise en place d'une opération de dépistage combiné VIH / VHC dans les officines de la ville de Marseille - DUMAS - Dépôt Universitaire de Mémoires Après Soutenance (cnrs.fr) - Accessed June 9, 2023, at Mise en place d'une opération de dépistage combiné VIH / VHC dans les officines de la ville de Marseille

(11) State of knowledge on hepatitis C and its management in dentistry.) Accessed 9 June 2023, at https://dumas.ccsd.cnrs.fr/dumas-01471020/document)(thsese)

(12) Roudot-Thoraval, F. (2002). Epidemiology of hepatitis C. médecine/sciences, 18(3),Article 3. https://doi.org/10.1051/medsci/2002183315

(13) GOOD PRACTICE GUIDELINES FOR THE PREVENTION OF HEALTHCARE-ASSOCIATED INFECTIONS OUTSIDE HEALTHCARE ESTABLISHMENTS PDF Free Download. (n.d.). Retrieved June 9, 2023, from https://docplayer.fr/2449392-Guide-de-bonnes-pratiques-pour-la-prevention-des-infections-liees-aux-soins-realises-en-dehors-des-etablissements-de-sante.html

(14) Blood exposure accidents-Aes. (s. d.). URPS Infirmière Paca. Accessed 9 June 2023, at https://www.urps-infirmiere-paca.fr/les-bonnes-pratiques/les-accidents-dexposition-au-sang-aes/

(15) Government of Canada, Canadian Occupational Health and Safety Council. (2023, April 5). CCOHS: Hand Washing: Reducing the Risk of Common Infections. https://www.cchst.ca/oshanswers/diseases/washing_hands.html

(16) Disinfection and sterilisation of medical instruments-Health Council. (n.d.). Retrieved June 9, 2023, from https://www.pharma-gdd.com/fr/desinfection-et-sterilisation-des-instruments-medicaux

(17) Hygiene and prevention of the risk of infection in medical and paramedical practicesConsulted 9 June 2023, at Haute Autorité de Santé - Hygiene and prevention of the risk of infection in medical and paramedical practices (has-sante.fr)

(18) AES and prevention - GERES. (n.d.). Retrieved June 9, 2023, from https://www.geres.org/aes-et-prevention/

(19) Blood exposure accidents-Aes. (s. d.). URPS Infirmière Paca. Accessed 9 June 2023, at https://www.urps-infirmiere-paca.fr/les-bonnes-pratiques/les-accidents-dexposition-au-sang-aes/

(20) State of knowledge on hepatitis C and its management in dentistry.) Accessed 9 June 2023, at https://dumas.ccsd.cnrs.fr/dumas-01471020/document)(thsese)

(21) Hepatitis C Educational Needs Assessment for Canadian Healthcare Providers (hindawi.com) .) Retrieved June 9, 2023, from Hepatitis C Educational Needs Assessment for Canadian Healthcare Providers (hindawi.com).

(22) Experimental hepatitis C vaccine developed in France I Reuters (n.d.). Retrieved June 9, 2023, from https://www.reuters.com/article/ofrtp-hepatite-vaccin- 20110804-idFRPAE77301Z20110804

(23) Chronic viral hepatitis C. Accessed 9 June 2023, at Microsoft Word - article38-09.doc (uca.ma)

APPENDIX

Appendix 1: Staff questionnaire

I) **Characteristics of the participating nurse :**

1. The service:

2. Age:22-30 years   31-40 years41-50 years   51-60 years

3. Gender: Male Female

4.Years of experience in current department :

0-5 years

6- 10 years

11-15 years

16-20 years old

21-30 years old

30 years to go

II) **general knowledge about hepatitis C :**

1. Have you taken part in any previous training on hepatitis C: Yes
No

2. Do you know what hepatitis c is?

Yes No

3. What agent causes hepatitis c?

Virus bacterium parasite other

If other, please specify.

4. How is hepatitis c transmitted?

By blood maternal-fetal sexual other

If other, please specify

5. How is hepatitis c transmitted in healthcare settings?

Needle stick Blood contact with healthy skin Blood contact with injured skin
Blood contact with mucous membranes

6. What are the complications of hepatitis c?

Cirrhosis Fibrosis Cancer other

If other, please specify
7. What can be done to prevent hepatitis c

Vaccination Single-use of medical equipment

Sterilisation of medical equipment other

If other, specify
8. Do you comply with the following preventive practices?

Yes No

Washing hands Wearing gloves Wearing a mask

Wearing a smock

Not recapping needles after use
9. Hands must be clean:
A. Before and after any contact with the patient and his environment

B. Before using gloves and after

C. can always be replaced by hydroalcoholic friction

D. Between two activities for the same patient

E. After accidental contact with biological fluids or contaminated objects

10. We recommend that you wear gloves:

A. If there is a risk of contact with blood or biological fluids of human origin

B. In case of risk of contact with mucous membranes and injured skin of the patient

C. Skin lesions on staff hands

D. The same pair of gloves can be used for the complete treatment of the same patient.

E. Unsoiled gloves may not be changed between patients

11. The overcoat:

A. Indicated where there is a risk of splashing a biological product of human origin.

B. Must be worn just before the gesture and removed immediately at the end of the sequence. care

C. Is changed between two patients

D. It must be worn by all patients in isolation, whatever thei illness

12. The mask is recommended in case of :

A. Risk of projection or aerosolisation of blood or products of human origin

B. Suspicion of lymph node tuberculosis during patient care

C. In the case of immunosuppression, unless the patient is wearing a mask

***III)* Assessment of attitudes and practices in relation to the risk of hepatitis :**

Please circle the correct answer(s)

1. What contaminating products do you handle?

*Linen stained with blood

*Puncture fluids

*Waste from genital sampling

*Biopsy products

2. what contaminating medical equipment do you handle?

*Hollow needles

* scalpels

*Solid needles

*athletes

3. Do you ever?

*Bend the needles

*Recap the needles

4. Protection and prevention :

Please tick the right answer

4.1. Do you wear personal protective equipment at work?

	Always	Often	Rarely	Never
Blouses				
Helmets				
Mud flaps				
Gloves				

4.2. Do you disinfect your hands with?

	Always	Often	Rarely	Never
Soap or bleach at 12° diluted 1:10				
70° alcohol or other antiseptic				

4.3. Do you disinfect the equipment? What do you use?

	Always	Often	Rarely	Never	
Heat					
Soap					
Bleach					

4.4. Do you disinfect the workplace? How often?

Product used:

Frequency:times/day.times/week times/month

4.5. Do you know the universal precautions for SEA? Yes No

4.6. Which of the following measures seem to you to be universal precautions?

- Do not recap needles

- Remove needles by hand after use

- Immediately dispose of sharps in safety containers after use.

- Wear gloves if there is a risk of contact with blood, biological fluids or soiled equipment

- Do not work in the department if you have skin lesions on your hand

- Wash your hands before and after each treatment

- Decontaminate soiled surfaces or objects with water only

4.7. What suggestions do you have for improving knowledge of HAEs and their prevention?

4.8. Is there any medical treatment available for acute hepatitis C? Yes No If so, what treatment?

4.9. Is there a vaccine available against acute hepatitis C? Yes No

Thank you for your participation

SUMMARY

Title: *Assessment of nurses' knowledge of chronic hepatitis C: epidemiology, modes of transmission, treatments and preventive measures*

Introduction: *Hepatitis C is a chronic infection of the liver caused by a virus that is transmitted mainly by blood. Nowadays, given the rising number of cases of chronic hepatitis C, these infections have become a cause for concern.*

Objectives: *To assess and enhance nurses' knowledge of HCV infections and help improve the management of patients with chronic hepatitis C and reduce its epidemiology.*

Materials and methods: This was a descriptive study directed at nurses working at the University Hospital of Gabès in 12 departments: women's surgery Our study focused on a population of eighty nurses working in general medicine, pneumology, cardiology, intensive care, dialysis, infectious diseases, maternity, emergency, gynaecology, paediatrics and male surgery, using a questionnaire. Our study focused on a population of eighty nurses. The survey took place in February and March 2023.

Results: *Our survey included a sample of 80 nurses working in the University Hospital of Gabès, with a sex ratio of 0.56, with a predominance of women (63%). Half of the population (52%) had no previous training in hepatitis C. With regard to general knowledge, the majority of nurses correctly mentioned that the agent responsible for HCV is a virus. With regard to preventive practices, our results show that the majority of nurses respected hand washing (86%), the wearing of gloves (82%), the wearing of masks (66%) and the non-capping of needles after use (86%). However, the majority of the population (61%) were unfamiliar with the medical treatment of hepatitis C.* *Conclusion:* *HCV infection is considered to be a major public health problem worldwide, because of its frequency and seriousness, linked to the high risk of progression to cirrhosis and cancer. At the end of our study, we can confirm that The population studied shows a lack of knowledge about certain details, which calls for awareness-raising and training to improve knowledge of this disease and thus improve care.*

Key words: *Hepatitis C, knowledge, nurses, epidemiology, modes of transmission, treatments, preventive measures*

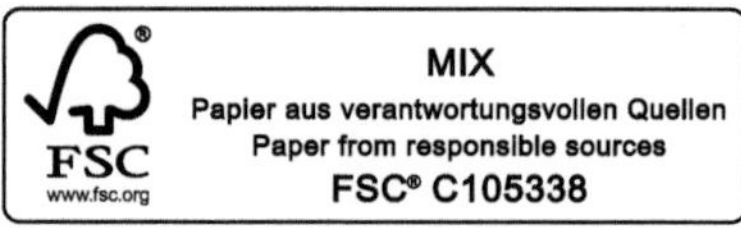

Printed by Books on Demand GmbH, Norderstedt / Germany